52 Things You Need To Pay Attention To When You Are In The Hospital

By Chioma L Okeke

About the Author

Chioma Okeke is a licensed Registered Nurse with a Bachelor's of Science Degree in Nursing. She is also an established writer and the founder of Choosing Nursing at choosingnursing.net where she provides additional advice and resources for nurses and nursing students. She prides herself in helping new nurses in successful transition into the nursing field. She is also a contributor for NurseTogether.com.

Special Thanks

Special thanks to my parents, my younger brothers for all their support.

Table of Contents

Preface

As a Registered Nurse with experience in the medical surgical and telemetry field, there is still an extensive need for education. Sentinel events in hospitals are still occurring and many individuals are fearful of being admitted to the hospital. This book was created to empower the reader. It was written as a tool for not only the patient and the family but also the nurse. The contents of the book are original and are taken from personal working experience.

CHAPTER 1

Labs

Whether you are in the hospital or if your loved one is in the hospital, it is important for you to have a general idea of your lab work. Granted, you're not going to know in detail what all of your lab work means or what should be done about it. However, it is important that you are aware of any abnormal labs. Abnormal lab work is a direct reflection of the illness you're currently experiencing. Improvement in abnormal lab work is a great sign whether or not your condition is improving. Depending on what you are in the hospital for, there will be specific and abnormal labs that correspond to it.

For example, if you are in the hospital because you had a heart attack, then there are specific lab values that may be abnormal. One of them is your troponin level which will be elevated. Troponin level or cardiac markers are enzymes your heart releases once there is damage done to it through a heart attack. It is important to know how high it is once you are admitted to the hospital and if it is trending downward. Granted, it is normal for you to have abnormal labs due to the illness you are experiencing, however, it is not normal for those abnormal labs to continue to trend upward as the days in the hospital continues to progress. This can be one reason why the physician has not yet discharged you. Your nurse will be the best person to know of your abnormal lab work. Your abnormal labs will also fill you in why the doctor is prescribing new medications, new orders, and or new or repeated procedures. Every single lab value is important, however, here are some specific lab values that are commonly more closely monitored than others.

K+ potassium 3.5-5.0

Na Sodium - 135-145

Troponin level -< 0.02

Glucose -70-110 mg/dl

WBC or white blood cell count 4.5-10 mcl

HGB hemoglobin

Men- 13.5-17.5 gm/dl Women 12- 15.5 gm/dl

Bun 8-20 mg/dl

Creatinine 0.6- 1.2 mg/dl

Understanding Lab Values

These are just a few of the critical lab values if you are on a general medicine floor. Your potassium level is very important because if it is abnormal, it can cause arrhythmias (changes in the rhythm of your heart). Your sodium level is important because when it is too low, it can cause seizures or confusion, especially if you are an elderly patient. Troponin level is usually monitored on a patient who comes in for chest pain or heart attack. A high troponin level is an indicator that the patient had a true heart attack. Your glucose level is very important because if it is too high, it can be an indicator of uncontrolled diabetes. And if it is too low, it can be extremely dangerous for the patient and cause them to be lethargic (very tired) and lose their level of consciousness. The white blood cell count is extremely critical because we look at this to determine infection. We don't look at this by itself; however it is a good indicator if someone is experiencing a new infection. Hemoglobin is important because if it is too low then we may need to give you a blood transfusion (infusing blood into your body). It may also explain why you feel so fatigued and may also show you have anemia that could be now diagnosed from being hospitalized. Bun and Creatinine are both important because if they are abnormal, it is an indicator of your kidney function. Your kidney function determines how well you are able to urinate and go to the bathroom. These are just a few of the really important lab values to be aware of.

Once again, keep in mind that the illness you or your loved one have will explain why they have higher labs when compared to others. For example, maybe you or your loved one is in the hospital for osteoporosis. Well, that would explain why your calcium level is low. And now the doctor is giving you new medications to help replace it. Either way it is important to be aware of the abnormal lab values at the *beginning* of your hospital stay.

CHAPTER 2

The Nurse

The nurse that you have is also something that you want to really pay attention to when you're in the hospital. Having a good nurse or having a bad nurse makes a world of a difference when you're being taken care of in the hospital. A good nurse will advocate on your behalf. A good nurse will be able to take things into account about you that the doctor is not aware of. A good nurse will be responsive to your needs. A good nurse can see things that will literally save your life when you are not even aware of it. Therefore, having a good nurse really matters.

Do not judge a good nurse by his/her age or how he/she looks rather judge him/her by their attitude and their caring nature towards you. Even if she is a brand-new graduated nurse, they still have the ability to care for you well because they have the desire to see you well. Take note if your nurse appears to be calm and confident. Having a bad nurse one day may or may not make that much of a difference. However, if you are in the hospital for longer than a day and you have a nurse that you in particular enjoy because of the level of care they provide to you, then there is nothing wrong with requesting to have that same nurse again.

Your nurse will usually be juggling many things at the same time but don't assume, it doesn't mean that he or she isn't competent. Instead, judge them by how they make you feel whenever you interact with them. Here is one question you can ask your nurse to see how competent they are and if they are credible. It's not their credentials, or what school because anybody can memorize that. Instead here is the question I want you to ask them:

"What is the plan for today?"

If they cannot give you a straight answer or if it doesn't line up with what is going on with you and why you're in the hospital, then I would pay more close attention to their behavior and then possibly ask to speak with the charge nurse privately.

"As a nurse, we have the opportunity to heal the mind, soul, heart, and body of our patients, their families and ourselves. They may forget your name but they will never forget how you made them feel"

-Maya Angelou

CHAPTER 3

Cleanliness

Paying attention to cleanliness should be an all-time high for you as a patient or for your loved one. A hospital that takes cleanliness important is a hospital that reduces infection rates, that lowers mortality rates, and that maintains clean environments for their patients. Some indicators that you can take note of that shows the hospital cares about cleanliness is by taking note if housekeeping comes to the room on a regular basis. Is there a housekeeper that regularly cleans the rooms, empties the trash and ensures the bathroom is clean? Cleanliness is also really important to disinfect the rooms before a new patient comes into that room. Otherwise, they may be leaving bacteria behind from the last patient which could easily make any immunocompromised patient sick once he/she moves into that room.

Hand washing is also an indicator of cleanliness. Does the hospital take hand-washing seriously? Does the staff wash their hands? Not just the nurse but the nursing assistant, the physical therapist, the doctor etc. Are there hand washing stations or hand sanitizer machines? Is it easy for people to wash their hands or is it something they have to search to find a place to wash their hands? These are all the questions you should take note of and ask yourself when you or loved one is in the hospital. It is a great sign if the hospital takes cleanliness seriously.

CHAPTER 4

Colored Signs Outside the Room

I will let you in on a secret when it comes to hospitalization and the hospital rooms. One thing that you will notice is that there are particular signs that are on the doors of the rooms before you enter inside. The intention of the signs is to let us as a staff to know the specific precautions we need to take before we go inside the room for that patient. These signs are indicators of what precaution and how contagious the illness the patient is having. You as a family member or friend visiting the patient in the hospital also should be aware of this sign. You should not just enter the room lightly if you see a sign on the door. The nurse is not required to tell you exactly what the patient has however he or she is required to tell you the type of precaution you should take before you enter the room. Here is the list of the color signs and what they typically mean. The type of colors may vary from hospital to hospital. However, this is the most common colors.

- Yellow sign - This sign is for contact precautions. With this sign, you need to at least wear the yellow gown and gloves before you enter into the patient's room to protect yourself.

- Green sign - This sign is for droplet precautions. This means you need to wear a mask on your face before you go into the room. Otherwise, you could run the risk of exposure through what you inhale. This means there is a room for exposure to whatever bacteria the patient may carry once you come within a 3 feet radius of them (ex: coughing, sneezing etc). However you wearing the mask prevents this from happening.

- Orange sign - This sign is for airborne precautions. This is also the most serious precaution you need to be aware of. The patient may have some kind of lung viral infection so it is very important that you cover your mouth and nose very well with the appropriate mask. This is much more serious and you MUST speak with the nurse before you enter the room. As the staff we actually have to be specially fitted with the appropriate mask before we enter into the room of these patients. The name of this type of mask is called an N-95 mask. As a visiting loved one, because you obviously can not be fitted for a mask, check with the nurse which appropriate mask you should wear before entering the room. One of the most common viral infections the patient may have with this sign of the door is tuberculosis. If a patient has a true tuberculosis infection, the hospital is required to notify the CDC.

As the patient witnessing whether it is the staff or loved ones coming in the room with these precautions is not something you should allow to affect you emotionally. These precautions are taken as more so also a way to prevent the bacteria itself from spreading.

Additional info: Methicillin Resistant Staphylococcus Aureus (MRSA) is a common strain of bacteria that can be acquired in the hospital or as normal flora (normal bacteria). As a normal bacteria, it can be present in your nose (MRSA in the nares). MRSA is strain of bacteria that has developed a resistance to certain antibiotics. It may not always cause harm to your body since it can be a normal flora. However if patients who are immunocompromised acquire it, it can have a very negative health consequences to them. Hence one reason why hand washing is so important.

CHAPTER 5

Your Medications

It is important that you are aware of what medications you are on. If you are watching over your loved one, it is important that you are aware of the medications they are on. The medications often will change from time to time or day to day when the patient is hospitalized. However, it is so important to be aware and take note of the medications.

Also, you must be aware of why the patient is receiving or why you are receiving that medication. Some patients will be on multiple medications but it's still important that you know what the purpose for each and every single one is. Medication errors can unfortunately be common so it is important that you also are proactive in your care while you're hospitalized. I would advise you write them all down so you can better keep track of them.

CHAPTER 6

The Timing of Your Orders Change

It is important to take note of the new orders that you or your family member is receiving while they are hospitalized. Examples of new orders can be chest x-ray, new IV fluids, new antibiotics, cardiac studies, etc. Take note that I did not only emphasize on the orders but also on the *timing* of the change in your orders. The timing means a lot. The timing could indicate you are getting better or you are getting worse.

For example, if you were just admitted to the hospital for pneumonia and it's been 5 days and now the doctor is ordering another new type of IV antibiotic and a more advanced chest x-ray (CT scan) that could indicate that your problem is actually getting worse and not better. Even so, your doctor should also be filling you in with any new changes in your orders. Timing can be the difference between you leaving the hospital in two days versus in two weeks. Therefore the timing of the changes in your orders matters.

CHAPTER 7

Edema or Swelling

If you or your loved one discovers there is new swelling or an increase of swelling in your arms and legs, this is a problem and you need to notify the nurse immediately. You especially need to notify the nurse if you are experiencing this problem and you have fluid running into your IV catheter lines. Swelling is not a good indicator.

You may also be prone to swelling because of the type of health condition you have, for example, kidney disease patients or heart failure. If you came in the hospital with swelling already then this is not the same, this is because of the condition you have. However if you have *new* swelling that was not there before, then this is a major concern. Either way, it still is something notable that the nurse and doctors should be aware of.

CHAPTER 8

Wheezing

Experiencing new wheezing and swelling can occur especially if you are receiving IV fluids in your IV line. Some patients who are experiencing fluid overload may be wheezing and not have swelling while others may have swelling without wheezing. Additionally, this is an urgent situation and needs to be addressed quickly with an appropriate intervention. If you or your loved one is experiencing wheezing that you did not have prior to coming to the hospital, then something needs to be done quickly about it.

Granted, you may not be able to listen to your own lungs or the lungs of your loved one, however, you can tell or hear wheezing often times while someone is just breathing. Do not ignore this sign. This can be addressed by ordering a chest x-ray and starting you on some kind of diuretic medication (which removes fluid from the lungs) to begin treating this problem.

CHAPTER 9

Your IV

When you or a family member is admitted to the hospital, we as nurses are required to insert something into your arm or hands in order to keep you hydrated and alive in case of emergency. This is called an intravenous catheter (IV). It is usually uncomfortable during the initial insertion However, it is not normal if it is still uncomfortable after it has already been inserted. The things you should pay attention to when it comes to your IV includes swelling, redness, and pain where the IV was inserted. These are symptoms you should not ignore and let your nurse know about it. This is not the same as a central venous line. This line is more critical and I would advise you to just allow the nurse to monitor and pay attention to the access of this line. Never manipulate any type of special IV line that's inside your neck, your chest or a PICC line in your upper arm.

CHAPTER 10

Your IV Line

If you are dehydrated or you are not eating, then your IV will be hooked up to a line and connected to a bag of fluids which will allow us to provide you with hydration in addition to nutrition until you are strong enough or well enough to drink fluids and eat on your own. If you notice that you are eating and drinking while you are still receiving IV fluids, then you should question or ask the nurse and doctor to see if you still need to continue with the line. It's important that you must have an IV line at all times when you are hospitalized because if an emergency occurs it will take us longer to administer anything you need during that hour and every minute matters.

CHAPTER 11

Your ID Band

Please make sure that anytime any staff member places an ID band on you or your loved one's arm, that it matches their name correctly. Don't assume that it is the correct ID band. Make sure if they ever change your ID band that it still says your name correctly. This is because there have been actual incidences where patients had the wrong ID band on their arm sometimes for even days! This means that they had the ID band with another name and birthdate of a different patient that is not them. This is a serious event that can be reported.

CHAPTER 12

The Doctor

Every doctor's role is different depending on the type of hospital they are operating in and their scope of practice. Some smaller hospitals only have one doctor to many patients. Most larger facilities have at least three or more doctors to one patient, not including their specialty doctor. These minimum three doctors usually include the intern, the resident and the attending doctor. The intern doctor is still learning and recently completed medical school. What they will primarily do is physically assess you and take notes of anything occurring with you. The resident doctor is the physician you will encounter the most who will write and intervene with new orders for you. The attending physician oversees all the doctors however delegates the majority of the responsibility to the resident physician.

Your doctor matters. What your doctor orders can literally save your life or if they are poorly educated, end your life. Fortunately that's one reason why the nurse is so important because even if the doctor writes the wrong order, the nurse is the one who actually carries out the order. The nurse is the one that will have to catch if there is an error in the order before carrying it out which is why the role of the nurse also matters. Your doctor will not spend as much time with you as your nurse however they can make the world of the difference during your hospital stay.

Depending on what you are in hospital for you will also have a specialty doctor. For example if you were admitted for having a heart attack you are going to have a cardiologist come and take a look at you. If you are admitted because you have kidney disease you are going to have a urologist come assess you. Here is a list of common specialty physicians that may also assess you depending on why you are in the hospital:

- Cardiologist

- Urologist

- Infection Disease Specialist

- Pulmonologist

- Neurologist

- Etc.

Every physician's role is different so you may find that one doctor is giving different feedback from what your primary care doctor is telling you. Be patient and trust they will come with a common plan for your diagnosis.

CHAPTER 13

Your Orders

Paying attention to your orders is important when you're in the hospital. The reason why you want to pay attention to all your order is to be certain that the orders that are being done to take care of you are correct for your condition. Of course you're not going to know exactly what all your orders mean. However, you have the ability to ask. Anytime you receive a new order or the staff informs you of a new change in your care plan, you should always ask them why it is being done for *you* specifically if they have not explained already. If they cannot address that question, then there is something wrong and you need to get clarification.

CHAPTER 14

Your Care Plan

Now, when it comes to your care plan, this is what the plan of care is for you in order for you to safely leave and be discharged from the hospital. The most ideal situation is at the start of the day, your nurse informs you of the necessary things to expect throughout the day. Also your doctor should make you aware during their rounds what to expect concerning your health for that day. However, there can be times when things may change or there may be updates in your plan of care. Typically, the doctor will inform you of the plans they have for you that day before it happens and why they are doing it. You as the patient as well as the family should always be involved in the plan of care. You must always make an effort in your care plan so you have the best outcome possible.

CHAPTER 15

Physical therapy

Sometimes when you become sick, it also affects your musculoskeletal health. This makes it difficult for you to walk or too weak to walk normally like you did before the sickness. Older patients usually have this problem worse when they are hospitalized. As a result, the physician should order something known as physical therapy where a licensed physical therapist will come to the room and perform exercises with the patient in order to strengthen their physical strength. Undergoing good physical therapy can be the difference between someone being discharged home as opposed to a skilled health facility. It is important for you to take a note of a new patient or your loved ones musculoskeletal health and see if they need to receive physical therapy so that there cannot be a delayed of being discharged home.

CHAPTER 16

Procedure Rationale

You would actually be surprised at the number of patients who undergo procedures or surgeries and still have no idea why they are undergoing it. Even if you ask the family members, they are still unclear as to what the procedure is truly for. So at times, you will see some patients asking questions concerning a procedure right before they have it done even though they signed a consent form.

It is extremely important that you as the patient or your loved ones are aware of not only the name of the procedure but why the procedure is done. Ask questions and make sure all your questions are clarified first *before* you sign the consent form. As the nurse, if we take notice that you are still unclear about the procedure, we are required to have the doctor come and talk with you again until you understand why you're having the procedure done. This will also help delay extended hospital stays.

CHAPTER 17

Your Room

Now, this is not applied to most patients. However, it is important to take note of the type of room you are being hospitalized in. The most important example of this is if you are in a negative air pressure room. A negative air pressure room also ties into the type of problem or condition you may have. However, it is important to keep the door closed as much as possible if you are in a negative air pressure room.

Some hospitals will have a double room where two patients are in the same room or a single bed room. Whether you are in a single or a double room it does not matter unless you are immunocompromised (see Your Roommate).

CHAPTER 18

Your Roommate

Now not all hospital rooms are set up so you would be paired with a roommate but some are. The charge nurse is responsible for settling you in a room that is appropriate for your health condition. If however you have a severely weak immune system then it is very important that you are not matched into a room with another patient who has an active infection. This can be very dangerous and cause further problems for the immunocompromised patient.

For example, if a patient has leukemia which is a form of cancer, it would not be wise for us to keep you in a room with a patient with a patient with pneumonia. This makes transmission of bacteria very easy and susceptible. Now of course you're not going to know nor is the hospital staff required to tell you what your roommate has a diagnosis of. However, if you know that you are immunocompromised, it is important to be certain the right precautions are being taken and placed for you. It may be best that you are in a room alone if this is the case.

CHAPTER 19

Your Nursing Assistant

Now some people actually don't take much attention to the nursing assistant but your nursing assistant can be just as important to your health or the health of your loved ones as the nurse is. The responsibilities of your nursing assistant involves handling your hygiene needs, helps to walk you, monitors your food intake and how much you're going to the bathroom. If your nursing assistant isn't taking note of these things or isn't paying attention to your hygiene needs, this can actually affect the type of information that is relayed to your nurse so that he or she can appropriately and effectively take care of you.

Your nursing assistant should always identify themselves to you at the beginning of the shift. Your nursing assistant will always have additional patients aside from yourself to take care of. Next to your nurse, your nursing assistant will usually be the one to answer your call lights whenever you need something. Your nursing assistant helps to assist the role of your nurse so they do not carry the scope or practice to do everything your nurse does. Here is a list of the duties your nursing assistant is responsible for:

* Help you to the bathroom

* Give baths

* Take care of your hygiene needs ex: brush teeth

* Record how much food you eat

* Record how often you went to the bathroom

* Walk you around the unit (if okay by the doctor)

* Notify the nurse of any new changes they see in your health

* Take your vital signs regularly

* Transport you to any procedures you may have

* Relay any information you want your nurse to know

Remember that every single person's role in your hospital care matters, so acknowledge each person and know that your nursing assistant matters too.

CHAPTER 20

A Hospital on Strike

I would honestly advise you if possible to try and not be hospitalized in a hospital during a time when they are undergoing a strike. This is because there is not as much order and care focus on the patients because the hospital is paying more attention to the strike. This can cause serious error, as well as life and death situations for the patients. Care can be delayed because of hospital strikes. The staff that would normally take care of you is out on strike and in replacement of them is outside foreign staff that is not familiar with the policies and procedures of the hospital you are residing in. Thereby creating more room for error. So if possible, I would strongly advise you to not be hospitalized or have your loved ones hospitalized in a hospital that is undergoing a strike.

Now the reason why hospitals go on strike or nurses go on strike is not simply because of financial gain or because the nurses are being greedy but it is truly because there are some very serious issues with the way the hospital is delivering care and no other measure of speaking up has been effective. It usually can take months before a nurse union decides to go on strike so it is not an overnight decision. Sometimes what the nurses will see is repeatedly happening is that the administration or representatives of the hospitals are budgeting costs that is affecting patient safety as well as nurse retention. Oftentimes hospitals with poor salaries for the nurses with high workload demands will not retain nurses.

As a result of not retaining these nurses, hospitals are filled with more newly graduated nurses as well as traveling outside nurses than there are permanent staff. The problem with this is less experience as far as nursing care and less nurses aware of that hospital's specific policies and procedures; which provides more room for error and higher risk to the patients. This is just one reason why nurses will elect to go on strike because at the end of the day, it's affecting the patients, whether on the strike or off the strikes.

CHAPTER 21

Your Vital Signs

Your vital signs are important. Your vital signs matter. Your vital signs are one of the greatest indications to us that there is something wrong with you even if you are not physically showing any signs. Now of course your vital signs will automatically not be the norm especially if you have pre-existing conditions such as high blood pressure or kidney disease. However, here are the normal vital signs and the range of abnormal vital signs that require some kind of intervention from us. You as the patient or the loved one watching your patient should also be concerned about these numbers. Take note of any abnormal vital signs you may have.

Blood Pressure	120/80
Temperature	98.6
Respirations	12-20
Pulse	60-100
Oxygen	93%-100%

* Pain is the 6th vital sign which is always graded from a scale of 0-10. Vital numbers vary differently for children.

Sometimes the patient will have adverse vital signs but they will not "feel" any symptoms or they will feel strange but their vital signs will not reflect any abnormal problems. In both situations there must be some kind of appropriate intervention. If the patient is having very low blood pressure (less than 90 systolic) with an elevated heart rate (above 100) this can be very life threatening and the patient may be showing signs of shock. Shock means that the body's organs are beginning to shut down and is trying to compensate by making the heart work harder. We have to respond to this immediately and delay in care can literally mean life or death for that patient.

If the patient's blood pressure is very high (ex: above 180 systolic) then the patient has a high likelihood of developing a stroke. A stroke can be life altering as well as cause permanent damage to the patient's brain. It is important to respond quickly to both extremes.

CHAPTER 22

The Color of Urine in the Foley Catheter

When you are hospitalized, some people will need to have something called a Foley catheter inserted into their bladder in order for us to measure the amount of urine they are producing, as well as the color, consistency, etc. All these factors are also indicators as far as the type of health condition or problem you are experiencing. If you notice a change in the color as opposed to the normal yellow as before or you notice there is no output coming out for several hours, then you need to let the nurse know. These are also signs that the nurse and nursing assistant should be aware of but it's good for you to pay attention to it as well.

The reason why the color also matters is because this is a sign the kidneys of the patient are failing or getting worse. The color of the urine is an indicator of damage to the kidneys. Sometimes however the color can be changed because of the medication the patient is taking. For example, Pyridum which is used to treat urinary problems can cause the color of the urine to change to orange. Here is a list of some of the common changes as well as normal in color that can occur with the urine:

- Yellow

- Dark Amber

- Brown

- Dark Yellow

- Orange

- Bloody Red

When the patient's the urine becomes bloody red, sometimes depending on the orders from the doctor, the nurse is required to begin irrigating or "flushing" the urine. This also helps to relieve any blood clots as well.

CHAPTER 23

Hand-Washing

Any good hospital will take hand-washing seriously just as much as they take doing surgeries seriously. Hand-washing is important because it prevents the transmission of bacteria that can be easily carried and distributed to the public, as well as to the patients that are already immune compromised in the hospital. Handwashing really does and can save lives.

If a staff member touches a patient with an active infection and then touches another patient with a weak immune system without washing their hands, they can transmit that bacteria to that patient which worsens their condition or even leads to death. You as the patient or the family member can take notice if the hospital takes hand-washing seriously by just looking around. Take a note if they have hand-washing stations, or hand sanitizer machines or if the staff washes their hands. All these things are signs that this hospital takes hand-washing seriously. Hand washing can be life or death for a patient.

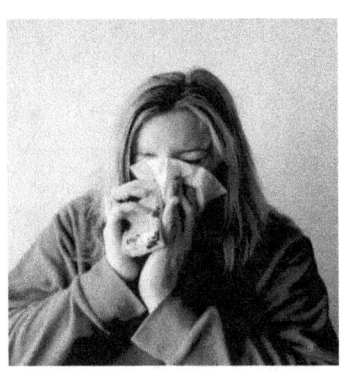

CHAPTER 24

Chest Tube

Not everyone will have a chest tube, however, chest tube placement occurs in patient with severe lung problems or patients who are gunshot wound victims. If you or your loved one ever have a chest tube, it is important to take note if the dressing site is clean with no signs of bleeding and if you ever have problems breathing or you feel short of breath to let your nurse know immediately by pushing the call light. Changes in your breathing is an even higher priority when you have a chest tube. The nurse will monitor the actual chest tube itself.

CHAPTER 25

Nasogastric Tube Placement

If you or your loved one is in the hospital and they have a tube going down their nose into the stomach, this can be one of two reasons. One reason can be for decompression which is to alleviate and/or remove contents in the stomach which may be one reason why you the patient or the family member has been vomiting and/or experiencing nausea. The nasogastric tube helps to remove the excess stomach bile accumulating in the stomach and goes into a special chamber.

The other reason is for nutrition. A nasogastric tube can also be inserted for feeding into the stomach. The number one thing that you as a patient or your loved one should be paying attention to is when the tube is no longer intact or pulling out farther than it was before. This is especially worse if the patient or loved one is being fed through the tube, because then, instead of the food going into their stomach, the food could go into their lungs which can cause them to aspirate. This is unfortunately a problem that occurs in some instances where patients have died. However some of things you can do to prevent this is to notify the nurse if the tube comes out, if the tube is noticeably longer than before. The nurse should be checking placement at the beginning of the shift to prevent risk for aspiration. Some patients who have a high risk for aspiration are:

- Elderly patients

- Infants

- Confused patient

- Bed bound patients

Aspiration can be deadly but it is also easily preventable. Special precautions should also be taken place when moving patients with nasogastric tubes.

CHAPTER 26

Watch Your Baby

If you have seen some stories on the news of babies being abducted from hospitals, it is true. This can happen and it is definitely a concern. If and when it occurs, we call it a Code Pink which means that a baby has possibly been abducted from the hospital. It is important that you as a new mother never take your eyes off of your new baby. If someone wants to do something to your baby, have them do it in front of you.

If you are having additional new medical problems and you need to go to another floor, then you would have to have a family member watch your newborn baby. Otherwise, you should never take your eyes off your baby, even if they are staff and have an ID badge on or are wearing scrubs. There was a recent incident where a baby was taken from a new mother and was told the baby was going to have a routine check. Unfortunately, the baby was actually taken to have a surgery that was performed on the wrong child. So if at any time, whether they are staff or not, whatever they want to do to your baby have them do it in front of you.

If your baby is sick and needs additional care for example on an NICU floor than this is different and you have to allow them to perform the necessary care needed to better the health of your baby.

CHAPTER 27

Oxygen

Sometimes, you or your loved one may need to be placed on oxygen from the start of your stay in order to help promote their health and make their condition better. The more oxygen you require, the more serious your problem is and can often equate to longer hospital stay. It's important for you to keep track of how much oxygen you or your loved one is receiving on a day-to-day basis. It's important to monitor if the oxygen amount is going down or if it's going up. If it's going down, that's a good sign that they are getting better and would soon leave the hospital. If it's going up or if they cannot take it off without having problems, that is a sign that they may need to go home with the oxygen or wait before they can be discharged.

CHAPTER 28

Speech Therapy

Some patients when admitted in the hospital have a problem swallowing that makes it difficult for them to eat or drink anything or sometimes, even talk clearly. There could be multiple reasons for this. One of them may be a stroke. However, is important that if they are having problems swallowing that their speech is assessed through the expertise of a licensed speech therapist. The speech therapist will come to the room and do exercises at the bedside in order to test how well the patient's speech is and if their diet can be advanced or needs to be regressed, as well as if they need additional new orders done.

CHAPTER 29

Blood Transfusions

A blood transfusion is when a patient receives donated blood into their IV line which goes into their bloodstream that will help improve their blood count. Patients are usually given blood transfusions when they have a low hemoglobin level (see Labs for the normal hemoglobin level). Before a patient can have a blood transfusion, we have to test their blood type, as well as obtain consent to be able to administer the blood. Please bear in mind that if you begin to feel hives or pain down your lower back area or extremely hot during the process of undergoing a blood transfusion, let your nurse know IMMEDIATELY because this means you're having some kind of negative reaction and the transmission needs to be stopped immediately.

In earlier times such as the 1980s, blood transfusion were even a scarier thing because the same precautions that are taken now were not taken thing. People weren't screened very well for health conditions such as hepatitis or HIV. This is not to say people were admittedly donating their blood knowing they had these conditions but rather they did not and they passed it on to someone else through the transfusion. As a nurse I personally have taken care of patients who have no history of hepatitis in their family nor no behaviors that contributed to it however they contracted hepatitis from a blood transfusion during that era.

Now better precautions are taken into place where transmissions such as this are extremely rare.

Here are few conditions where you or your loved one may need a blood transfusion:

- Sickle cell anemia

- Low hemoglobin Count (severe anemia)

- Severe blood loss from trauma or surgery

CHAPTER 30

Post-Surgical Complications

There are many types of surgeries one can undergo while they're in the hospital with a potential complication for each but I will not list them all here. What you need to understand is that there is always a potential for complications after surgery. Your nurse should do a good job of taking note of any sign of this type of complications. However, here are some things that you can be made aware of or pay attention to:

- Difficult breathing

- Bleeding on the dressing site

- Changes in your temperature

- Numbness

These are just a few of the more common complications after a type of surgery or procedure that you should pay attention to and make your nurse or doctor aware of right away.

Some of things you can do to be proactive with your care so you can be discharged sooner is that soon as your nurse gives you the okay, begin walking around the unit frequently; even if you are in pain. This will help increase gastric motility in your abdomen so that you don't develop an illeus or need pain medications long term. An illeus is the inability of your bowel systems to move normally. The sooner you begin to do this, the better it will be for you.

CHAPTER 31

Your Pain Medications

I understand that the pain that you or your loved one experience will be very uncomfortable and you will desire to be medicated with as much pain medications as possible. This is very normal. However, your goal should be to slowly not have to need the next medication or as many pain medications as before. You should expect for the doctor to discontinue your IV pain medications. The reason you don't want to stay on pain medications for too long is that it can cause potential problems. Some of these problems may include; respiratory depression, constipation, confusion, etc. You want to try and come to a point where you only need to take oral pain meds just as you were before becoming hospitalized. Here is a list of some common names of IV pain medications you or your loved one may receive:

- Dilaudid

- Morphine

- Morphine drip (pain pump)

- Toradol

CHAPTER 32

New Signs of Infection

Take note of the key word that I used in this section which is "new". Many patients that come to the hospital are coming because they have an infection. However, if you are in the hospital for something unrelated to infection such as chest pain and then you begin to experience *new* signs of infection, this is something you need to pay attention to and make the nurse and or doctor aware of. Here is the list of signs that would indicate you have an infection. Also take note that just because you have one or two of these signs, it doesn't automatically mean that you have an infection, but it may need to be monitored more closely.

• Fever

• Sweating

• Redness

• Swelling

• Pus (greenish or yellow)

These are just a few of the symptoms that may indicate you have an ongoing infection. However, we will usually confirm it with the appropriate labs as well.

CHAPTER 33

Your Risks

You need to know ALL the potential risks that you or your family member could have with the procedure the doctor is having done on you or ordered for you. There are many patients that undergo a procedure and then develop a risk and state that they were not aware that such was a possibility, even though they signed the consent form which states all the risk on it. Make sure that you know the risks for all the procedures that are being done to you. The risks will always vary depending on the kind of procedure you are undergoing. Here are some examples of common procedure risks:

- Nausea/vomiting

- Paralysis

- Stroke

- Loss of limb

- Death

CHAPTER 34

IV Push Medications

Remember that earlier in this book, we discussed your IV catheter and the importance of having an IV line and to make sure that it is in a good condition? Well, one of the things that we do through your IV line is give you medication. Not just pain medications but other types of medications as well. There are different ways that we give these medications and some of them involve where we directly push the medications with our hands using an IV push syringe into your IV line. However, there are some medications that should never ever be pushed into your IV line. This can cause serious problems for you as a patient or your loved one. Here are two medications that should never ever be pushed on a regular medicine floor without special precautions in place:

- Dilantin (safe to give as IVPB)

- Propofol

If you see this happening, stop the nurse and ask if you can talk with a charge nurse about the medication you are receiving via IV push. Also note that only a registered nurse should be giving you any type of medication through your IV line.

CHAPTER 35

Your Heart Monitor

Depending on how advanced the hospital that you're staying in is, you may have a basic heart monitor that is required to always be on your chest at all times so we can monitor your heart rhythm. Not all patients need to be on a heart monitor. This is typically only for patients with some type of heart-related diagnosis. The heart monitor also allows us to respond quickly in case you are having sudden changes to your heart that needs to be addressed immediately. If you notice that your heart monitor is not working correctly then make your nurse aware or any other staff member aware so they can address the issue right away.

CHAPTER 36

Your Linen

Your linen is important. You need to be certain that it is clean when it is newly placed on your bed. Your sheets, blankets, pillow cases etc have to go through a thorough washing before they are placed on your bed. Strange stains should not be ignored and should be exchanged for a new clean linen. There are special bins in your hospital room where you place the dirty linen. This important so that the housekeeping can regularly bring new clean linen for you to use.

CHAPTER 37

Fall Risk

The risk you or your loved one has for a fall is something the hospital staff does not take lightly. Hospital Falls can lead to other major problems such as trauma, skin bruises, injuries, sometimes even as critical as a stroke. Having a fall can also lengthen you or your loved one's hospital stay. Some things you can do in order to prevent a fall from occurring include:

- Wearing the appropriate socks,

- Wearing the appropriate arm bands

- Asking for help before you get up or get out of bed

Being in the hospital forces you to be more dependent on others however know that it is okay to ask for help before you get out of the bed, *every time.*

CHAPTER 38

Unusual Sudden Pain

Pain is never a good sign but having unusual sudden pain can be serious. One of the examples I mentioned earlier was feeling sudden lower back pain during a blood transfusion. Another great example of unusual sudden pain is severe chest pain. Severe chest pain is not something that the staff should take lightly and it needs to be treated immediately for the sake of your own health. If you ever have unusual sudden pain, you need to push the call button and immediately let your nurse know.

CHAPTER 39

Your Bowel Sounds

One of the things that we as the nurses assess or pay attention to is your stomach especially if you are having some type of bowel problems such as a small bowel obstruction (a blockage that inhibits food from passing through your intestines). When you are not experiencing any sounds coming from your stomach area, this is an indicator that we need to hold any food and not allow you to eat at this time. This can happen for hours, sometimes days or even a longer duration of time and usually by this point, we have to place you on some type of nutrition through an IV line. However, what you need to understand is when you have no bowel sounds, you're not able to eat at that time therefore it is important for you to abide by any orders telling you to abstain from food.

CHAPTER 40

Signs in the Room

Not only are there signs outside of the room but there are also signs inside the room that indicates specific ways we need to handle your care. These signs are very important for your safety, as well as the safety of your loved ones. Examples of the signs may include:

- Blind in left eye

- Unable to hear

- No food by mouth

Is there any certain care about yourself or your loved one that you feel all the staff should know before or while contacting them? Then let the nurses know about it so they can place the appropriate sign above your bed.

CHAPTER 41

Bed Sores

One of the major concerns many family members have for their loved ones when they are in the hospital, in particularly elderly patients, are bed sores also known as pressure ulcers. Pressure ulcers occur in patients who are either bed-bound or have an inability to move positions in their bed independently. As a result, they are dependent on the nurses and nursing assistants to keep turning them on a regular rotation. The reason why they develop pressure ulcers is because they cannot turn on their own which therefore places pressure on those areas of their skin which can affect the tissue and the bone. Frequent and severe pressure ulcers is a sign of poor care provided to the patient and should not be addressed immediately. The normal rotation of turning patients is usually a minimum of 2 hours to up to 4 hours.

CHAPTER 42

The Bed Type

You should also pay attention to the type of bed you or your loved one is sleeping on particularly if they are at risk of pressure ulcers. It is usually necessary to place these patients on a special mattress bed to even further reduce the risk of pressure ulcers. Smaller hospitals may not be able to afford such beds. This is why it is even more important to keep them turned regularly.

CHAPTER 43

Your Discharge Date

Take note of your discharge date. Typically, the norm is for you to only be in the hospital for about 2-3 days. However, this can vary incredibly depending on what you are in the hospital for (for example trauma, medical emergency). You want to pay attention to your discharge date, not just because of the cost of each day (that's important too) but if your discharge date is being prolonged or pushed back, make sure you clarify with your doctor why this is so. It can be due to your illness, maybe it's not getting better or there could be other issues that's indirectly prolonging your hospital stay (for example; no staff available to complete your procedure). Be aware of these things and get to the root of the problem.

CHAPTER 44

Your Discharge Teaching

Once you or your family member is discharged from the hospital, you MUST take note of every single thing that your doctor, as well as your nurse is teaching you upon discharge. Every detail is very important. Not heeding to all the instructions could potentially cause you to return to the hospital soon. It can cause you further complications or new problems as well. So you want to read through everything once you get home, as well as listen to everything the nurse/doctor tells you.

CHAPTER 45

Procedures

There are a multitude of procedures patients undergo in the hospital. Both nursing, as well as medical procedures performed by the doctor but the specific kind of procedure I am referring to is any procedure that involves penetrating any area of your body. This can go all the way to a heart catheterization procedure to something much smaller such as insertion of a Foley catheter. Procedures that involve penetrating any area or orifice of your body are more important to take note of because they all have one potential thing in common: risk of infection. There is always a risk of infection which could lead to worsening conditions, longer hospital stays and unfortunately, even death sometimes. If you or your family members notice any new signs of infection (redness, fever etc) AFTER having any type of procedure done, notify the nurse IMMEDIATELY. If he or she does not believe you or take you or your loved one seriously, speak with the charge nurse, the doctor, a patient advocate until someone believes you. It can literally mean life or death if it's not treated immediately.

CHAPTER 46

Call Light Responsiveness

Whenever anyone is admitted to the hospital, in order to help reduce new medical emergencies, falls, etc, everyone has a call light inside their room which should always be kept within arm reach. A call light is similar to a control attached to the bed that patients can press to turn on lights, TV and most importantly, ask for help from the nursing staff. The use of call lights should be reduced through hourly rounding which is when the patient is checked on at least once an hour. However, the call light is still provided so the patient's needs can be attended to if necessary between those times.

How well the staff attends to the call lights is another sign of the type of care provided. If the norm is for call lights not to be responded to for several minutes even up to an hour or more, then this is concerning especially if the patient is having a true medical emergency and no one is responding to them. Now there are a few exceptions because some patients actually abuse this privilege which takes the nurse off the attention of the patient that really needs their help but generally call light responsiveness is a great indicator of quality of care.

CHAPTER 47

Language Interpretation

It is important that every facility has a kind of access available for language translation especially when there are patients who are not fluent in English. There are usually two methods used for English translation in a hospital facility. One method is to use someone in the medical staff to translate sensitive information to the patient. Using family members to translate is usually avoided because of the sensitivity of the information given to the patient. Another method is phone translation. There are phone services that allow the patient to listen and the staff to speak and on other side of the line is a medical translator to accurately translate to the patient. Always ask for an appropriate form of language translation if the patient or your loved one does not speak or understand English.

CHAPTER 48

Medication Patches

There are some medications that are administered to patients on top of the skin or *topically* in either a patch form or adhered to the skin. The most important fact about medication patches to really take into account is that they are for severe pain. Leaving medication patches for pain for an extended amount of time than prescribed or not replacing these patches (for example, putting new one on without removing the old one) can lead to very severe problems including death.

Strong analgesics can cause symptoms such a respiratory depression, confusion, and death. Long term use must be monitored with great precautions. One of the necessary precautions that should be taken especially when it comes to any analgesic is monitoring the patient's blood pressure. Strong analgesics have the ability to slowly lower the patient's blood pressure to dangerous levels. It's understandable to want the patient's pain level to be treated but however if they are not really in true severe pain, a medication patch can have more adverse effects than positive.

One particular drug that is commonly administered and that you want to be mindful of is Fentanyl. If not used properly, it can lead to life threatening problems. Fentanyl is usually placed on the skin for 72 hours then it is rotated to a different site with a new patch. You must always remove the old patch before replacing the new patch as well as not leaving it therefore extended periods of time. Sometimes patients with cancer can be prescribed Fentanyl patches for their severe extended pain. However Fentanyl patches should not be taken lightly.

There was a story of a mother who had a young boy and she was on Fentanyl patch for her pain. She was on the patch because she had chronic pain. Then one day, her son was also complaining of pain but she did not have any pain medication to give to him at the time. Not knowing the severity of the patch, she placed the patch on her son where he was stated he had the pain. Within a few hours they boy's pain was improving however the mother left the patch on her son overnight. The next day she woke up to discover that her son had died in his sleep. You must be careful with medications especially medications for pain and only take what you are prescribed and do not administer it to others without a prescription.

Another kind of medication patch to take note of is Nitropaste. Nitropaste is not a patch but more so of a paste that is adhered to the skin for patients who come in with complaints of chest pain. The Nitropaste can treat the chest pain as well as lower high blood pressure. Nitropaste is changed every 24 hours. The previous administration should always be removed prior administering the new one. It can be very effective for chest pain but if not closely monitored, it can also cause very low blood pressure.

Additional Info: Lidoderm is also another common medication usually administered in the hospital to patients with very severe pain. It is usually placed 12 hours on and 12 hours off.

CHAPTER 49

Seizure Precautions

If you or your loved one is in the hospital and has a history of seizures, aside from administering the correct medication, there are also other precautions that need to take place. One of the main precautions is placing seizure pads against the rail/sides of the bed. This is because if or when the patient does have a seizure, they will not injure themselves by hitting their body against the sides of the bed. If you or you know your loved one is having seizures, make sure their bed is padded well to prevent injury.

CHAPTER 50

Medical Restraints

Sometimes when the patient comes into the hospital, they are already so confused that they may become a danger to themselves or others that they need to be secured in the bed with restraints. This can also occur when they have already been hospitalized and there are changes in their mental status hence causing them to be a danger so they need to be placed on the restraints. If the doctor orders it, it is absolutely necessary that you as the loved one acknowledge it. NEVER ever, remove the restraints without first asking the nurse. I know this can be hard sometimes because this is your loved one and you know them well but during this time, you have to respect the orders. There have been times where the family *while* in the room with the patient will remove the restraints and they turnaround or go to the bathroom only for the patient to climb out of bed, fall or even DISAPPEAR. And yes, this is while the family member is in the room because they underestimated their ability. Patients shouldn't be on restraints for very long periods especially if the patient is becoming more alert but while they are on, you as the family or friend visiting must respect the orders for their own safety, as well as yours and those around you.

CHAPTER 51

Teamwork

Depending on the type of unit, this may or may not truly play a role in how well the care that you're receiving is. However, it can for other places. Teamwork is best noted through observation; seeing how the nurses, the staff cooperates with each other. Teamwork is important because it also shows quality of care. Teams that work cohesively together have happier patients and more accountability. Teams that work together are focused on obtaining GOALS that benefits everybody especially the patients. Therefore teamwork matters when it comes to receiving excellent patient care.

CHAPTER 52

Your Surgery

Before you have your surgery done, even if you are currently in the hospital as you are reading this, there are a few things I want you to take note. First and foremost, RESEARCH the physician who is having the surgery done on you. The Internet is so accessible to us now so it's easy to find this information. When you research the physician, see how long they've been a physician, what kind of reviews they have or if they have multiple counts of legal cases against them. The staff is not normally going to confide in you if a physician does not have the best success rates (and yes, there are working doctors like this) so it's your due diligence to take note of this. If you see a red flag, ask questions, trust your gut and request a different physician to perform your operation. In regards to your surgery, you also want to look up if it is the norm for the hospital you are in to do your procedure. Do they have the appropriate equipment, as well as good patient success rates? Once again, you can learn this information by simply doing your research, as well as asking questions and exploring the hospital's website for more information.

Acknowledgements

Thank you for reading this book! I hope you found all the information very valuable to you and I would encourage you to take this book with you every single time you or your loved one is in the hospital. The amount of information is too vast to collect it all in one sitting. Share this book with a friend or a loved one. It could potentially save or even change their lives for the better.

Sincerely,

Chioma L. Okeke RN, BSN, PHN

www.ingramcontent.com/pod-product-compliance
Lightning Source LLC
Chambersburg PA
CBHW071821200526
45169CB00018B/509